Contents

Sex Science:

21 SIZZLING Secrets That Will Transform Your Bedroom into a Sauna!

By C.K. Murray

Sex.

We all know what it is. Even if we don't always talk about it. Even if it's so taboo in some cultures, that to merely *hint* at its existence could be sinful.

Sex is the thing that people do behind closed doors. It is the 'steamy' scene in a movie; the twitch of the muscles, the curl of the toes. It is the lip gloss and the nail polish and the skimpy, sultry allure of a body bordering on nude. It is the chiseled frame of muscle; the outline of a stark figure with a dark past. A fundamental part of the human experience.

Sex is normal.

It is the act that consecrates, that desecrates. A means of communication, a vehicle for passion, for reassurance. An outlet of anger, of caring, of fear and fury. It is a maelstrom of emotions, tossing covers and heaving pillows; the battering of sweat-slicked bodies in dark rooms, beneath sheets *screaming* to be released.

Sex is hot, sex is weird, sex is something and nothing— sometimes meaningless, sometimes everything.

It is known by a million names. Some are vulgar like "fuck" and "bang" and "screw" and "pound" and "shag." Some people "make love" and others "hook up." A college kid is simply trying to "get laid," while a close couple wants nothing more than to "get intimate."

When it comes to sex, there is always an agenda.

It doesn't have to be evil or hidden. But it can be. Sex for one, is rape for another. A good time to you, is a bore to me. Consensual or forced; ambivalent or invested. We all want something out of it—perhaps selfishly, perhaps not. What doesn't stop us, makes us stronger. What doesn't give us pleasure, only makes us bolder.

Or does it?

Virgin or seasoned, sex is never far away. In porn, in movies, in shows and salacious novels—intercourse is omnipresent. No matter what you may call it, or how you may appraise it, sex is an intrinsically human act. Men and women, women and women, men and men, or multiple members of each gender—having sex can take *all* forms and functions.

And it is in these many forms and functions, that the *fun of fornication* becomes something more. Beyond this very carnal act, a very *real* science has emerged…

Hot Head—Your Brain on Sex

From the moment you wake up, to the moment you go to bed, roughly 100 million acts of sexual intercourse will have occurred. And in almost all of these cases, the brain—that complicated grey thing between our ears—is even more active than those *other* things between our legs.

See, when people engage in intercourse, the body is obviously doing something drastic. We are all aware, to some extent or another, that our organs are in contact, and that it is this movement, this friction, that creates the feeling of pleasure that ultimately *erupts*.

But what about the other movement, that crazy wild dance, that is occurring in our neural pathways?

During intercourse, the brain is awash with activity. All thoughts, feelings, and bodily sensations we experience are associated with specific nerve cells under activation. Neurons are cells that shoot chemical and electrical signals through the brain's wiring. Their various shapes and paths deliver specialized functions, such as remembering how to skewer your hips, or how to tighten your abdomens in an attempt to hold off orgasm.

Neurons like to chatter. When they communicate, they fire impulses across gaps called 'synapses.' These messages are electrical by nature but turn chemical when crossing synapses. This chemical form is called a neurotransmitter. Once the neurotransmitters reach the other neuron across the synaptic gap, they are converted back to electrical form.

These neurochemical changes take place in a primordial, mammalian part of our brain, the limbic system. It is this 'system' that is common to all mammals, and controls nearly all our bodily functions. The basic role of the limbic system is to keep us alive and reproductive. Thus, it repeats what is pleasurable and avoids with is painful. It is the catalyst for our emotional, impulsive, desire-based drives—especially sexual ones. It makes us fall in love, it makes us lustful—it makes a once torrid affair turn dry and forgetful. The limbic system has been around for many, many millions of years, embedded beneath the more 'rational' segments of our brains.

Basically, the gadgetry of the human mind is always at work. One of the most important pieces of the limbic system circuitry is called the reward pathway, and it is this 'pathway' that plays such an important role in behavior. Because the reward pathway connects to other parts of the brain, it is tightly bound to our five senses.

When we have sex, the senses tell us that what we are doing feels nice, and the neurotransmitter dopamine is released. This important neurotransmitter gives us the feeling of pleasure that the brain remembers. As a result, memories of the pleasurable experience are gathered and the reward pathway reinforces the behavior. Dopamine causes us to repeatedly seek the behavior, even when other practical impediments show up. In many cases, it is the excess of this chemical, dopamine, that may lead to addiction. Imaging of sex addicts' brains has made this clearer.

It is amazing how carnal and one-minded the limbic system drives can make us. Take for instance, studies done on rats. In one such experiment, a starving rat is placed on one side of a grid with an electric current dividing that grid. Across the pain-producing grid, there is food on the other side. Although the food may be there, and the rat may be starving, the rat will not cross to the other side, as it knows that the electrical current will cause incredible agony. However, when an electrode is planted in the rat's reward pathway, the rat will happily cross the electrical threshold, merely to press a lever known to excite the reward pathway. Thus, the rat will blindly rush to tap the lever, simply for the resulting pleasure, even though getting to that lever causes pain, and even though the rat should be more focused on alleviating its extreme hunger. In many of these experimental setups, the rats will continue to rush across to tap the lever, till the point where they die of either starvation or electrical trauma.

As crazy as this sounds, sometimes things aren't *much* different in humans. Consider for instance, another phenomenon, called the Coolidge Effect. To understand this phenomenon, we must first acknowledge an important truth: no mammals, humans included, are monogamous. We may be 'socially monogamous,' forming bonds and unions that ensure familial units, but we are still drawn to new sexual possibilities. This is because our genes want as many avenues for potential reproduction as possible. Staying sexual monogamous is, more or less, putting all our eggs (or sperm) in one basket. Simply put, social custom and evolution will oftentimes butt heads.

Because humans are not sexually monogamous by nature, maintaining interest in a single partner can become very trying. The Coolidge Effect describes this very problem. Before even looking at these attitudes and behaviors in humans, it's easy to see them in our close relatives, monkeys. When male monkeys are paired repeatedly with the same females, those males engage in copulation less and less frequently. Even when the females are injected with hormones to keep them continually 'horny,' the males quickly lose interest.

Of course, the entire equation changes when *new* females show up. Despite how lethargic and sexually disinterested males become with the same females, the instant new females appear on the scene, the males' libidos skyrocket. It pretty much all comes back to the neurotransmitter dopamine. As mammals copulate with the same partner, less and less dopamine stimulates the reward pathway.

However, when a new partner—a new stimulus—appears, dopamine spikes.

Dopamine flooding the reward circuitry is capable of overriding perceptions of fullness or satiety. Our rational brains may give us a million reasons not to, but many times, it's the emotional, ravenous reward 'brain' that wins the battle. Our genes tell us to follow what is good and pleasurable. This explains many situations, especially one at the dinner table.

Ever been totally *stuffed*, but then dessert appeared? And suddenly you were able to wolf down pieces of a glistening chocolate cake, despite being "full"? Well if so, you have a basic understanding of how the reward circuitry can take precedence over our minds and bodies.

But now this begs a new question. What would happen if you and your partner did *not* have sex as frequently, and the dopamine levels did *not* decrease as they do in the Coolidge Effect? Well, this *might* sustain the union between you and your partner by preventing excessive sexual satiation—but not for long. Unfortunately, because orgasmic sex would be occurring less often, the emotional bonds would weaken. It would reach a point where authentic affection would dwindle as contact and interaction fell off. In the end, affectionate would only manifest as a narrowly goal-oriented behavior: to reach orgasm.

When we consider the Coolidge Effect and the countless other hurdles life throws our way, it's no wonder that so many couples end up in therapy or counseling for their sexual woes. Of course, there *are* coping strategies for a depleted sex life. Many couples introduce novelty to their lives and change their routines, doing things they never once considered. This may include acting out fantasies or engaging in role play; trying BDSM, fetishes, and orgiastic experiments; or simply, changing the position, place, or circumstance of sexual activities.

Still, none of these coping strategies will work if the involved partners are not open. Without an honest dialogue about wants and needs, partners will never achieve the sustained sexual satisfaction they seek. As a result, many relationships may fall apart, compounded by the intersection of rationality and emotionality. Emotional and desire-based drives that go unfulfilled will eventually be rationalized, and struggling couples will find reasons to part ways.

And in some cases, addictions may ensue. If extreme measures are taken to chase the dopamine 'high' associated with sexual pleasure, some people may fall far, far into the pits of a most powerful and pervasive dependence…

The Power of Porn: How Instant Access to Sex is Reshaping Our Neural Networks

Nowadays, sex in all its shapes and forms is merely a mouse click away.

The pornography or "adult entertainment" industry is one of those profit monsters that continues to operate in numerous media forms. In 2007, global porn revenues were thought be around $20 billion, with $10 billion coming from the U.S. alone. However, the Free Speech Coalition estimates that both global and U.S. porn revenues fell by half between 2007 and 2011 due to—you guessed it—the internet. In 2008, over 40,000 websites distributed pornography, and roughly 75% of them offered free material, usually as a means to lure in viewers to paid subscriptions.

With all the free porn online nowadays, it's no wonder that the words "sex addiction" and "porn addiction" have entered the public lexicon. Although many experts are slow to recognize such conditions as actual disorders, the tides are shifting. Many studies have shed light on the attitudes and behaviors of so-called porn addicts, but now, new research is showing that the very brains of these individuals are similar in activity to those of drug addicts. A study at Cambridge University revealed that compulsive porn watchers exhibited similar activity in their reward pathways when watching porn as alcoholics did in seeing adverts for booze.

As more studies pour out, the clinical psychological and medical communities are taking notice. In the latest edition of the Diagnostic & Statistical Manual of Mental Disorders (DSM-V), sex addiction and porn addiction are all categorized under the same disorder. Although they are not called "sex addiction" and "porn addiction," the conditions are provided for. As of now, the so-called "Hypersexual Disorder" can only be diagnosed in those age 18 and older:

- *Over a period of at least six months, a person experiences recurrent and intense sexual fantasies, sexual urges, and sexual behavior in association with four or more of the following five criteria:*

1. *Excessive time is consumed by sexual fantasies and urges, and by planning for and engaging in sexual behavior.*

2. *Repetitively engaging in these sexual fantasies, urges, and behavior in response to dysphoric mood states (anxiety, depression, boredom, irritability, etc.).*

3. *Repetitively engaging in sexual fantasies, urges, and behavior in response to stressful life events.*

4. *Repetitive but unsuccessful efforts to control or significantly reduce these sexual fantasies, urges, and behavior.*

5. *Repetitively engaging in sexual behavior while disregarding the risk for physical or emotional harm to self or others.*

- *The person experiences clinically significant personal distress or impairment in social, occupational or other important areas of functioning associated with the frequency and intensity of these sexual fantasies, urges, and behavior.*

- *These sexual fantasies, urges, and behavior are not due to direct physiological effects of drugs or medications, or to ManicEpisodes.*

Specify if:

- *Masturbation*

- *Pornography*

- *Sexual Behavior With Consenting Adults*

- *Cybersex*

- *Telephone Sex*

- *Strip Clubs*

- *Other:*

The problem with this "hypersexual disorder" is that it only applies to those who are 18 or older. This is problematic because many of those most vulnerable to the effects of porn compulsion and addiction are younger teenagers. With the inculcation of sexual content in today's modernized societies, kids are being exposed to porn quicker than ever before. With their developing brains, already wired by technology, they are *extremely* susceptible to addictive habits.

Heterosexual males especially see the impossible, artificial standards set by porn websites. Given the highly cosmetic nature of porn actresses, young male teens unconsciously begin to compare 'real-world' women to those in the sex videos. Love and lust have become further dissociated. The porn once used to relieve sexual tension and prepare for real sexual relations is now *replacing* those sexual relations.

So then what can we do?

How can sexual partners keep their relationships lively and sustainable? In an age of instant sexual gratification, how do we manage our frenzied reward pathways and lead lives that are both fulfilling and functional?

Well, the answer surely isn't simple. But there *is* an answer. And it all begins with understanding. That is, understanding how men and women think. No matter your sexual preference, researchers are finding that men and women approach the act of sex with very different mindsets. Emotional, physical, and psychological factors all collide to create the strange and varied world of *sexology*.

The Birds and the Bees: Reconciling Differences between Male and Female Sex Drives

Let's be honest, men and women have always thought differently. Sometimes the reasons are clear-cut and sometimes they seem virtually inexplicable. Regardless of the scenario, science is beginning to uncover these differences, and bring great light to many 'stereotypical' beliefs. Let's take a quick look at how men and women differ in attitude and behavior when it comes to sex. By noting the disparities in sex drive, both genders can learn to readily adapt to situations that may cause… *tension*…

Men Think More about Sex and Seek It More Frequently --

Surveys show that the majority of adult men under the age of 60 think about sex at least once a day. Meanwhile, only about 25% of women think about it as frequently. As men and women age, they fantasize less, but men will still fantasize twice as often. Research also shows that men report more spontaneous arousal, spurred on by more consistent and varied fantasies. This is true beyond the heterosexual realm. Gay men also have sex more often than lesbians at all stages of a relationship.

When it comes to self-gratification, roughly two-thirds of men say they masturbate, and about 40% of women say the same. Prostitution is still mostly a phenomenon of men seeking sex with women, rather than the other way around. Even when it comes to vows of chastity, the trend continues. About half of nuns admit to sexual activity and over 60% of priests state that they have done the same. Men generally report more partners.

Women Have a More Complicated Sex Drive

Sometimes *women* don't even know what turns on women. One such study at Northwestern University had interesting results. When erotic films were shown to gay and straight men and women, the gay and straight men responded as expected. Both gay and straight men expressed sexual arousal to the images of male-male sex and male-female sex, respectively. Devices attached to their genitals corroborated these feelings. However, when it came to women, ladies expressed most arousal by male-female sex, but their genitals showed the same level of arousal to all images: male-female, male-male, and female-female

It is then no surprise that women's sexuality is more plastic. They are more capable of same-sex relationships, even if they don't choose to engage in them. Many lesbians have also reported sex with men. Studies show that women are more likely to call themselves bisexual and report sexual orientation as a choice.

Women Take a Different Route to Getting 'In the Mood'

Women want something more like a romance novel. They need a certain contextual feeling before engaging in sex. Studies show that women have more imagination than men and want to take a more roundabout, emotion-laden route to intercourse. For men, the route is pretty short and straight.

Basically, women want to talk first, connect first, then have sex, experts say. Men use sex to express their intimacy. For women, sex is more of a consummation of all the intimate moments that have come before.

Women's Sexuality Affected More by Culture

Renowned gender and sexuality psychologist, Baumeister, asserts that the literature is highly convincing when it comes to the effect of culture on the female sex drive. Some of the pertinent points revealed are:

- Women's attitudes and willingness for various sexual practices are more likely to change over time

- Women who regularly attend church are less likely to be promiscuous. For men, it does not matter

- Women are more influenced by the attitudes of their peers when it comes to sex

- Women with higher education levels are more varied in their history of sex acts. For men, no correlation

- Women are more likely to be inconsistent in their expressed values about sexual behaviors and their actual behaviors.

Women may be more affected by the power structures of patriarchal societies. Moreover, women are hard-wired to choose their partners carefully, since they are the ones that end up tending to the baby. They're more likely to choose a man with resources and a man who shows the ability to last—as both these qualities are important in supporting a child.

Women's Libidos are Less Affected by Medicine

If men's sex drives are more affected by biology than women's, it's no surprise that men are more susceptible to drug effects. Pills for erectile dysfunction and testosterone are quite useful for men. When it comes to women, however, drugs aren't doing much. Although testosterone works in women, it works much less effectively than it does in men.

One comprehensive survey has revealed that though 40% of women report some sort of sexual problem—typically low sexual desire—only 12% reported being bothered by it. As a result, many argue that formulating a drug to solve the 'problem' should be the last resort. In short, men and women should strive to renew their libidos through natural means first.

Women are Less Likely to Orgasm

Speaking of libidos and sex drives, men typically have a lot less trouble when it comes to… well, cum. On average, men last for 4 minutes—from entry to ejaculation. If women do orgasm, it usually takes around 10 to 11 minutes. Among couples, ¾ of men say they always orgasm, compared with 26% of women. Female partners can accurately note when their male partners orgasm. Men, however, think that their female partners reach orgasm 45% of the time, as opposed to the actual figure of 26%.

This is due to several reasons. Women may want to please their partners, and may feign orgasm. Also, the female orgasm is often difficult to achieve. It is not uncommon for some women to never orgasm. Reaching this pleasurable moment often takes a lot of self-exploration, and sex experts urge women to be persistent. Sometimes, the use of a vibrator is critical in 'hitting the spot.'

And speaking of 'hitting the spot,' sometimes it really, quite literally, is about hitting the spot. That is to say, the "G-spot."

MEN, Pay Attention! The Science of the "G-spot"

Chances are, you've heard of the G-spot. For years, the clitoris was believed to be the only way to trigger a **female orgasm**. And even as men everyway clamored to understand the location and power of this mysterious spot, the task was far from easy. Then, in the 1980s, the gynecologist Granfenberg found a new location in the vagina with a different type of tissue. Sexologists soon termed this new area the "G-spot." Stimulation of this area was said to deliver a very powerful kind of pleasure, one that could even elicit female ejaculation. Multiple times.

For the sake of exactitude, the G-spot is usually described as an "erogenous zone," analogous to the male prostate. It is bean-shaped, spongy, and the tissue of the paraurethral gland. It is roughly the size of a quarter and feels rougher to the touch than the surrounding tissue. When stimulated properly, it will swell quickly with blood.

In order to locate this special spot, one must go about two inches back from the vaginal opening inside the front of the vaginal wall; the front is the same side as the woman's belly button. The best way to get to the spot and master it is to face the woman while she is on her back. Insert your index or middle finger into the vagina as far as it goes without too much pressure. Then crook up the finger, and slide the fingertip along the top of the vagina until an area is found that is rougher than the rest of the vaginal wall. This slightly ridged area is the "G-spot," and touching it usually causes a woman to react with surprise or pleasure. Working it right may even get some women to have multiple orgasms.

It should be noted that not all women receive stimulation from the G-pot. Some may report discomfort or displeasure. Still, exploring the vagina may afford an opportunity to discover another pleasure region. After all, all women are different. If your partner is stimulated through the G-spot, do so by rubbing it with your crooked finger. Remember, don't be disappointed if you've tried everything and it doesn't work. You may find that women enjoy G-spot stimulation more during their 30s. As the estrogen levels go down with age, the vaginal lining becomes thinner and the G-spot is easier to reach.

Another way to stimulate the G-spot is through dildos that are designed specifically for the task. They will typically have a certain width, hardness, and curve. And speaking of curve, penile stimulation is often the most naturally stimulating, but the most difficult. However, for those who have penises that curve upwards, the task is made *a lot* easier.

The only way to hit the G-spot in the missionary position is to prop the woman's hips up with pillows. This allows for the right angle and can be facilitated by the woman contracting her pelvic muscles. Strengthening these contractions is critical for G-spot stimulation and can be perfected through Kegel exercises.

Of course, hitting the G-spot alone will not turn one from a novice to a master of the carnal. And let us remember, in the bedroom there is never just *one* master. Partners should strive to please one another so that the pleasure is shared. If one person is receiving all the 'goods,' the other person is likely to feel unsatisfied. And the relationship will sour. Now that G-spot stimulation is better understood, let's cover one for the ladies…

How to Give the Perfect Blow Job

Men will tell you, few things compare to a good blow job. In fact, some men may even prefer oral sex over vaginal. The beauty of a blow job is that it features a unique power dynamic. On one hand, the man is thrilled to see his lady submissive and placating, bringing his flaccid organ to a rigid rise. On the other hand, the woman is equally empowered by her ability to 'command' her man's most private muscle. Although some woman may be averse to giving oral sex, it is always worth a shot. The act is less about getting a man hard and more about the emotional and sensual connection. Obviously, if done right, it *will* get a man hard—but this is merely the destination. The real fun is in the journey.

Every man and woman will take to blow jobs differently. Some men want it slow, some want it quick. Some partners may opt for deep-throating while others may have desires that include the licking and sucking of the testicles over and over. Ladies, when it comes to your man, find out what he likes. And don't be afraid to simply ask. A simple, sexy "You like that?" or "Feel good?" can go a long ways in pleasuring the both of you.

That said, there are certain unspoken rules to follow when giving a great blow job. And in following these rules, what becomes most important is not what the woman should do, but what she *shouldn't*. Here's what *not* to do if you're looking to get the most out of oral sex with your man. Don't:

Avoid Eye Contact

They say the eyes are the window to the soul, and this shouldn't be surprising. When a woman is looking at her man, she is showing that she is receptive to his feelings and desires. If a woman doesn't look at her man during, he will likely think that she doesn't enjoy it, and this will kill the mood for both of you. If that connection isn't there, it might take much longer for the man to get hard. In the end, the man will be unsatisfied and the woman will feel incapable.

Hide Enjoyment or Pride

During a blow job, a woman should show some degree of positive emotion. If she doesn't actually enjoy the act, at the very least, she can be excited in knowing that it will prepare a man for vaginal sex—and thus her pleasure. Think about the experience of giving pleasure, of your man's groans and encouragement, of the way he breathes and heaves as you stimulate his penis like nobody else can! Take pride in your ability to sexually arouse your man—in the fact that he is sooo turned on by you. Remember: don't think of a blow job as a servile act that does nothing for you. YOU are an integral part of it, and feeling that soft organ turn rock hard in your mouth should get your blood pumping!

Ignore the Balls

Some women may be turned off by the thick, 'forestry' nature of a man's testicular region. Of course, a small bit of ball hair won't hurt you, but most women won't find it exactly enjoyable either. If your man likes his balls pleasured, you can always compromise. If he promises to keep them clean and trimmed, you'll play ball. When it comes to working the testicles, try different things.

Flicking the tongue, slurping, sucking, and even trying to fit them in your mouth are all good options. You can also use your hands to massage, knead, flick, or even squeeze those things! If you get really comfortable around that region, you might even find yourself working the taint or anus. When it comes to the balls, though, communication is key. Men don't always like women playing rough with their drooping tenders—so ask, explore, and find out what works for him! Who knows, maybe you'll get a kick out of watching those things jiggle.

Always Let Him Make the Move

Some guys will be pretty up front about what they want. They might bluntly ask you if you'll give them head. Others may gently steer your head downward, or give it a nudge; and others still will outright grab your face and shove it in. Depending upon your relationship and degree of comfort, it's always good to mix things up. Especially if you enjoy giving blow jobs, don't be afraid to initiate. Instead of waiting for your man to grab you and get it started, choose to work your way down there yourself. Maybe give him a devious grin and slip your hands in the pants. Perhaps slink downward, saying nothing with your mouth but everything with your eyes and lips. Or if you're *really* an upfront gal, grab the reins and command: "Take off your pants."

Forget the Hands

A good blow job will usually use the hands as an extension of the mouth. Grabbing firmly at the base with a little pressure will offer great stimulation and serve as a point of leverage. Using saliva while rotating the hand and changing pressure, speed, and length of stroke is a great tactic that will keep the man guessing, grunting, and heavily engorged. Twisting the hands in opposite directions, clockwise and counter-clockwise, moving them up and down the shaft—these are all techniques that should be tried and discussed with your man. Some guys might simply prefer a one-handed jerk.

Remember, your hands can also go to task caressing the man's stomach, chest, hip area, and inner thighs. And don't forget yourself! If you've got a free hand, nothing feels better than stimulating yourself while you stimulate your partner.

Go Too Fast

Go with the flow and be mindful. Don't think of other problems at work, with the kids, with friends, or other obligations or momentary concerns. If need be, put the clock where you can't see it, turn off your phones, and focus solely on the experience. Foreplay is like prebaking the oven, so don't hurry it. Unless this is some kind of quickie or time constrained fantasy, take time and have fun with a little 'preparation' before the actual penetration. Try: little breaks, hair pulling, licking, kissing, caressing, stroking, and even incorporating toys or lotions or stopping to change the music or adjust the mirrors. All of these things will increase the duration and allow more pleasure to build. In the end, the climax will be worth the wait!

Be Boring

Giving a blow job is a sensual experience not a mechanical process. This ain't an oil change. If you aren't changing up the rhythm and variety, you are likely to get tired pretty quick. And so is your man. Instead, challenge yourself. See what maneuvers or motions elicit the most reaction from your guy. If you get tired or uncomfortable, change position. Go from ass on your knees to kneeling if he's standing, 69ing, laying down on the bed as he stands, etc. Also, try not to vary too quickly. Sure, you might want to cover what you know your man likes, but that doesn't make you go about it like a checklist. The more you two engage in oral sex, the more organic it will all become.

And the more options you will think up!

Forget Saliva

Just as friction for women can be uncomfortable when they're not wet enough, it can also be tough for men. Sure, not every man will want an extremely sloppy blow job, but the other end of the spectrum is worse. Repetitive spitting, spit strings, and drooling will help to lube up the penis and will make the blow job that much easier. Easier to do, nicer too feel, and more pleasing for both—what's to lose? If a woman is averse to choking or gagging, she can simply repeatedly suck and spit. It might also help not to swallow while giving a blow job, so that saliva accumulates. If the woman likes, she can save the swallowing for the finale.

Overuse Your Teeth

Some guys like a little teeth grazing or nibbling on the balls… some don't. The truth is, men are surrendering their precious penis to your mouth, and the thought of teeth hitting their dick too hard is a thought that scares them. If using some teeth, be sure to open up the jaw. Sex experts recommend treating the dick like lipstick by rubbing it all along the lips and smothering it. Then, slurp and swallow like a creamsicle. Some women like to press it against the cheek before popping it out. This is a *huge* turn-on to many guys.

Run Away When He Cums

Assuming your man is clean, there's nothing to fear from cum. That is to say, there's nothing to fear that can endanger your life. Sure, some women like the taste and the look and the smell, and others are absolutely disgusted. When it comes to ejaculation, women who enjoy swallowing may have always enjoyed swallowing or may have learned to. Some women can tell when the man is about to blow because he gets a certain "O" face or makes a certain contract or utterance. The penis will reach its hardest state at this point.

When it comes to what to do with the ejaculate, women will run the spectrum. Obviously, some will swallow—if not for their partner's pleasure, for their own. Heck, some women *always* swallow. Other women may be okay with the semen going inside their vagina. Many may simply want cum on their breasts, tummies, or hair. They might rub it in, let it lie, or lick it off their fingers. Again, this all varies from woman to woman, man to man. Some men might not even like ejaculating on their partner; others will relish it.

If a woman can't even stand being around cum, but wants to try, think of it this way. Cum is the culmination of all that hot, naughty pleasure. It's the man's way of saying, you own me. You dominated my cock and made me blow. You, and you alone, made me cum like I did just now. Some women may view semen as a sort of reward for their efforts, and the look on the man's face as he catches his breath might just make their day. Cum is the man's body saying, "Oh baby, baby."

But cum is just the end. The most important part, of course, is everything leading up to it. And when it comes to everything leading up to it, cumming should be the last thing on a couple's mind. If you or your partner is having trouble with cuming too quickly, there are certainly things that can be done. Some are simple, some a little more complicated. But *all*, when used in tandem, can contribute to improved duration beneath the sheets.

MUST-KNOW Techniques for Lasting Longer

Lasting longer in bed is important to everybody's sex life. If it feels good, and is good for you, why wouldn't you want to prolong it? That said, making sex last longer while not compromising the experience can be a tall order. When it comes to increasing duration, men are the most anxious. Premature ejaculation and early ejaculation are common problems men report. By employing the following strategies men can not only further please their partners, but they can feel good about themselves in the process:

7 & 9

Don't know what this means? Similar to methods outlined in the Kama Sutra, the 7 & 9 technique is essentially a stroke-based method used to delay ejaculation. Basically, you start with 7 fast in and out strokes, followed by 9 slow ones. It's a good rhythm for women too and keeps the sex fresh and sustainable.

PC Workout

No, no, this doesn't refer to logging onto your personal computer and watching porn. The PC muscles, or pubococcygeus muscles, are the ones that stretch between the anus and urinary sphincter. By contracting and releasing these muscles, men can drastically improve their self-control for when the heat of the moment arrives. If you don't know how to work these muscles, simply practice stopping your urine flow in the middle of peeing. Doing several sets of 10-15 repetitions per day should be enough. Squeezing those muscles will promote strong blood flow to the penis and stimulate mental stamina as well.

Slow it Down, Change it Up

If you're nearing climax, alter your speed, or try a different position. Don't go jackhammer pace all the time. Learn to rotate your hips and undulate. Come in from slightly different angles and experiment with different twists and jerks. Go deep then shallow, shallow then deep. You can even try rubbing the head of your penis sensually near the labia. Because vaginas are loaded with nerve clusters, your partner will still find this pleasurable. Also, don't always focus just on the penis. Remember to nuzzle, and kiss, and caress. Fondle the clitoris and grope the breasts. If need be, close your eyes and cut off the visual stimuli. This might just save you from climaxing.

Medication

To date, there are roughly 20 different medications for premature ejaculation. Tablets and oral strips help to regulate neurotransmitter levels in the brain and thus increase blood flow to the penis. When using medicine, one may experience dry mouth, drowsiness, and other more severe symptoms. As always, stay in contact with a physician if you decide to go the medication route.

Master the Squeeze

Squeezing or applying pressure can aid a man in maintaining an erection. Make a tight ring with the index finger and thumb around the base of the erect shaft. This will help keep blood flow to the engorged penis. Also, try applying pressure to the underside of the head. Thirdly, press on "perineum," the area between the anus and the base of the testicles. This will delay the flow of semen and help stave off ejaculation. It's similar to holding the nostrils closed when about to sneeze.

When it comes to holding off that final blow, an understanding of the sexual response can also help. Researchers William Masters and Virginia Johnson divided the human sexual response cycle into four stages: excitement, plateau, orgasm and resolution.

In the excitement phase, an erotic physical or mental stimulation leads to sexual arousal. The penis will vacillate between being flaccid and being partially erect. The plateau stage occurs next, a period of sexual excitement prior to orgasm in which pre-ejaculatory fluid is typically secreted. During the orgasm phase, the plateau phase concludes and a quick cycle of muscle contractions happens in the lower pelvic muscles near the anus and main sexual organs. This wave of sexual pleasure occurs alongside the production and release of semen. Finally, the resolution stage calms the muscles and decreases blood flow to the penis. This phase must end before a male can undergo the previous stages all over again.

Of course, in order to *truly* perfect stimulation and extend duration, one must learn the truth about the male and female bodies. Because there are countless opinions and voices, it's sometimes hard to separate the science from the nonsense. In preparing for a bedroom of sultry, sexy fun, one would be wise to enter with the right information.

So let's dispel the myths.

12 Myths that are Killing Your Sex Life

Every area of science and study is plagued by myths. Pseudoscience rears its ugly head whenever it can, if not for the simple goal of self-preservation. Ignorance begets ignorance; stupidity continues to spread. For the sake of clearing the air, let's look at some of the common myths when it comes to sex and sexology:

Men Think about Sex Every 7 Seconds

This one is a little preposterous. This would mean thinking about sex virtually all day, as often as we are breathing. Some studies have shown that roughly 40% of men think about sex between a couple times a week to a couple times a month.

Menopause Effectively Ends a Woman's Sex Life

A comprehensive 1994 survey of U.S. sexual habits found that roughly half of women in their fifties have sex several times a month. Although hot flashes, pains and other disturbances may make a woman temporarily unable or unwilling to have sex, there is no direct link between menopause and sexual drive. Menopause does not have to spell the end of sex.

It's All about Penis Size

Sure, some women may enjoy men with larger packages, and some men may enjoy women with certain vaginal qualities. At the end of the day, though, it all comes down to emotional and physical compatibility. The average man is roughly 5 and half inches erect, and research shows that the size and shape of the organs mean less than the psychological connection.

As they say, "it ain't what you've got, it's how you use it."

It's Impossible to Get Pregnant When on Your Period

Conceiving during menstruation may be improbable, but it's not impossible. Once inside a woman, sperm can last up to a week, waiting for an egg. Ovulation can occur quickly after, or sometimes during, the bleeding phase of a woman's cycle. As they say, *never say never*.

Single Men Have More Sex than Married Men

A 2006 study by the National Opinion Research Center found that husbands have sex as much as 400 percent more often than single men. Married men are also more likely to receive and give oral pleasure. Not to mention, married *women* enjoy more orgasms than their single counterparts.

Doctors Can Tell Virgins from Non-Virgins

Women may worry about this, feeling as if the gynecologist is somehow gaining insights into their private lives. Well, this is *not* the case. Even under intense magnification, determining a virgin cannot be done accurately. Because all hymens have holes, it is not that simple.

Semen is Chock Full of Calories

Semen is comprised of water, vitamin C, calcium, magnesium and other nutrients. It also contains the sugar fructose. However, the calories are very limited. Interestingly, in a 2003 North Carolina State University study of 15,000 women, researchers found that women who regularly swallowed (one or two times per week) had a significantly lower occurrence of breast cancer over a ten year period than did those who never swallowed.

Women Don't Like, or Watch, Porn

While its' true that the adult entertainment industry is geared toward men, women certainly enjoy more than a peep from time to time. About a third of women report having watched porn and more than 10% of men report never having watched it.

For incorporating successfully into relationships, men and women should agree on content that suits both their needs. They should also supplement with toys, fantasies, and other varied activities. Porn is not simply "a guy thing."

Men Can't Have Multiple Orgasms

Sure, guys can only produce and release sperm so quickly and frequently, but that doesn't mean a man can't experience multiple peaks of arousal during intercourse. Women can prolong this by pinching the head of a man's penis when he is nearing climax. By then focusing on another part of his body, or simply allowing him to 'cool off,' women can essentially play puppet master.

Repeatedly doing this, will bring a man close to ejaculation multiple times, ultimately building to one heck of a crescendo.

How devious!

Women Reach their Sexual Peak at 28; Men at 18

It's true that men's testosterone levels peak at about 18, but hormones are only one ingredient in the sexpot. Meanwhile, women have no set peak. It's sort of like when people say, "you're only as old as you feel."

So stop thinking your libido is dwindling, and go out there (or *in* there) and get down to the get-down!

You Know What They Say About Guys With Big Feet…

What? They spend more on shoes?

Although the same gene influences the development of the penis and toes, the length of one does not predict the length of the other. In several studies of penis length and foot size, no correlations were found. These studies relied on researchers handling the genitals, contrasting with self-report studies where men are more susceptible to misreport.

Great Sex Should Come Naturally

First off, let's not be selfish. Sometimes people have sex to create intimacy, to fall asleep, to reduce stress, or for the purpose of procreation. Sometimes, one partner will be doing the pleasing while another time, the other partner will be the one placating.

In a 2009 NSSHB study, data revealed that roughly 30% of women reported pain the most recent time they had sex and about one-third were not adequately lubricated. On the men's side, 1 in 5 guys reported feeling that they ejaculated too soon.

Other studies have echoed the reality of less-than-perfect sex. Among satisfied couples who have regular sex, sex is considered "very good" at the most, one fourth of the time. Couples call it "good" roughly half the time.

For those who think sex should be amazing every time— get real. No thing in life is incredible every time. Like many aspects of living, an enjoyable sex life can take some work, some patience, and some conscience. And if you want to take your sex life from mediocre, to good, to great, to *otherworldly*, you've got to make the right plays…

21 SIZZLING Secrets That Will Transform Your Bedroom into a Sauna!

When it comes to 'spicing' things up beneath the satin sheets, think novelty, not frequency. If you or your partner is complaining of a less-than-stellar libido, of a sex life staler than black mold, simply trying to have sex more often is not going to do it.

If you want to *do it* like the wild animals you know you are, then you need to do *this*, first. That is, do *all* of this, first… or at least some:

Ladies: Panties ON

In the bedroom, torture is sometimes pleasure. Lingerie is one of those tantalizing things that can play with a man's mind to no end. Instead of stripping nude immediately and doing the deed, enjoy some deliberation. Keep the panties on while you stroke and caress, and allow the anticipation to mount. It will make the end that much sweeter.

Coital Alignment Technique

Missionary is the least effective position for reaching female orgasm, but if it happens to be the position of choice, there are several things you can do. A woman should have her partner move his entire body up roughly two inches. This will bring the man's pubic bone at a rest atop of the woman's so that the base of his penis presses on the clitoris. This position is good because it ensures continuous stimulation of the clitoris throughout, which just might bring on an orgasm.

Pre-romp Rinse

Hop in the shower for a little kiss and grope. Whisper words to one another, expressing all the naughty things you two have in mind. Stroke and rub, but not too much. This will get both of you hot and ready—and then it's on!

Stand-up Sex

Having a quickie against a wall can be totally unexpected and exciting. Try to do it spontaneously, pulling at each other's clothes and leaving kisses and saliva spots up and down the body. Or, if you're feeling extra dirty, let the penetration come immediately. It might just take both your breaths away!

Give and Take

Happy partners will learn that equal satisfaction doesn't always mean equal work. Sometimes, the man wants to take control. Other times, the woman wants to be the one who is dominant. Just as a woman may find the power of her partner incredibly intoxicating, men also love to see their lady grab the reins. Some women love to ride their man, as he lies unmoving, enjoying the sweet, sweet undulations of her hips, abdomens, and vaginal muscles. Mix it up and set your boundaries. All this give and take might just bring on the perfect orgasm.

Dragon Breath

This one is a cool little technique that will make sex all that more fiery. It can be used before or during lovemaking, especially if orgasm is not being reached. Simply take rapid, rhythmic and shallow breaths through the nose. By doing this for several minutes with the mouth closed, the blood will become oxygenated and sexual energy will skyrocket.

Back, Baby, Back

Known as the sacrum, the vertebrae in the small of the back is a surefire erogenous zone. It is located right above the buttocks and is full of nerves that connect straight to the genitals. By lying on your stomach and having your partner press on the sacrum with the palm, it's almost impossible *not* to get aroused. Just try it!

Talk it Out

It's important to be open with your partner, but not critical. Try encouraging when he or she is doing something you like. If need be, gently guide your partner's body to the location or in the motion that you like. If discussing sexual problems in general, save this conversation for a quiet place outside the bedroom. And most importantly, create an atmosphere of caring and tenderness. Don't equate sex with love. Maintain emotional and physical intimacy first. If you are trying to force this kind of intimacy when all you have is sex, chances are your relationship won't sustain—without some serious changes.

Sunrise Sexing

Morning sex is better for your health and mood. Like a coffee, it will get you energized for the day, but unlike a coffee, it won't have the dreaded crash. Moreover, sex in the morning is great for men, because the male testosterone levels are peaked around this time. Men will last longer and finish with more potency. For an especially intimate moment, have sex to the sun rising. Also makes for a great lazy Sunday wake-up!

Handy Time

The hands are very sensitive. Place the tip of the tongue on the webbed area at the base of the fingers, then slowly slide the tongue and lips along the side. Like the inner ear, these nerves are starving for more attention—and will love it when they get it. Sucking the fingers will turn up the notches even further!

Chuck the Clock

Forget the notion that sex should be done at night. Find time in your busy schedule and make it happen. Some people enjoy having sex right after work, at evening time. It makes for a nice little 'happy hour' and can help you pull through that last stretch of tough tasks at work. Nothing like a little nookie to look forward to…

Missionary Maximized

If you really like the missionary position, there are cool things you can do. To ensure the deepest penetration, pull the woman's knees up to the chest, then spread them barely wide enough for penetration. With the woman's calves on either side of the man's back, the female can support his weight on the backs of her thighs. As the man does his thing, the woman can rock back and forth for optimal mutual stimulation.

The Eye of the Beholder

Visual stimuli is very important when it comes to enjoyable sexual experiences. Keep the lights on and the eyes open. Use mirrors or video cameras. Enjoy doing naughty things that you can see from all angles. Relish the movements of all body parts, from all conceivable perceptions. Sometimes you'll have to remind yourself that it's actually *you* doing it!

Fabrics and Colors

A survey of 2,000 British adults by retailer Littlewoods found that partners with purple bedding or furniture had 3 and a half "intimate encounters" weekly. Those with grey had the least amount. Beyond just colors, bedding fabrics also contributed to differences in encounters, with silk sheets getting play just over 4 times per week. Duvets, on the other hand, elicited the least sexual encounters.

Red Hot Passion

The *Journal of Personality and Social Psychology* found that men were more likely to say they wanted sex with a woman in red and would spend more money on her. Although other studies support this, men surveyed report that red clothing does not make them perceive a woman as more intelligent or charismatic. Simply more attractive.

Slow-Mo

It's called "peaking" and essentially it means assuming a slower-than-normal pace, with the exact intent of building slowly to an incredible peak. Going too fast can be painful if not boring, because it dulls the mind and does not allow for feelings of intimacy or connection. By going slower and longer, partners can enjoy the rhythm, tension, and muscular contractions that make sex so amazing.

Mindfulness

Meditation is key. Studies show that men who are able to practice yoga every day can as much as *triple* their duration during sex. Basically, the body of research indicates that stretching and isometric holds in yoga increase core strength and pelvic muscle control, thus allowing guys to stave off orgasm longer.

Shower Sex

Doing it in the shower can be amazing. The water, the heat, the lubrication—it can be very mind-reeling. Start by throwing down a rubber shower mat so none of you fall while in the act. Then, get in one of two positions. You can (1) have the woman face the shower wall with one foot on the far corner of the tub while you stand behind her. Or, you can (2) face each other and have her hook a leg around your waist, as you rest a hand on the shower wall. Just be sure not to get too sudsy with the soap. Latex is damaged by soap, which can cause breakage.

Self-Preparation

If there isn't much time for foreplay, do it yourself. Let's be honest, you know your body best, so when it comes to getting ready, you might just want to be the one to do it. Watch each other as it happens and maybe even speak a few naughty words. Sooner rather than later, you both will be ready to delve head-first into intercourse.

Massage

Erotic touch and massage is indispensable. Set the mood with a warm room and candles, and nice scents like lavender. Massage deeply along tension areas such as the shoulders and lower back. Vary between gentle touches to deeper squeezes. Sometimes silence is golden; other times, asking questions like "right there?" or "how does that feel?" or "you like that?" is the way to go.

Master the Tongue

This one applies to both men and women. When it comes to oral sex, suction is only one part of the equation. Flatten the tongue and pretend to be licking an ice cream cone. Stroke up and down and from side to side. Vary the pace and frequency. Flick the tongue. Allow saliva to pool. Work the clit, the vagina—the whole thing. Work the shaft, the balls, the head—the whole thing.

Oral sex can be *very* pleasurable.

And in the end, isn't that what it's all about? If you or your partner or *partners* are struggling to fulfill sexual desires, it's time for changes. The main thing is pleasure. It doesn't have to be a strictly carnal pleasure—but there should always be some relation to feeling *good*. Intimacy with your partner should please you. Connecting emotionally should make you feel good. Having sex, or kissing, or sharing in a favorite activity, or merely being in each other's wordless presence—it all should make us feel good. Pleasure is a complex thing that humans can barely even define at times, but the fact remains: if you're having sex, if you're allowing your organs to connect with another person but you aren't pleased by it—then what *exactly* are you doing? Sometimes, pleasure is pain, anger, explosion; some nebulous mix of emotions that we can't describe but can certainly feel.

Sex is *a lot* of things, and as humans with that thing called the brain, it's up to us to figure it out. Or, at the very least, cum a little bit closer.

A Special Note:

Thank you for reading *"Sex Science: 21 SIZZLING Secrets That Will Transform Your Bedroom into a Sauna!"*

And may you continue to live healthily and happily.

Sincerely,

C.K. Murray

Other works by C.K. Murray:

1. *The Blood Pressure Diet: 30 Recipes Proven for Lowering Blood Pressure, Losing Weight, and Controlling Hypertension*

2. *Coconut Oil Cooking: 30 Delicious and Easy Coconut Oil Recipes Proven to Increase Weight Loss and Improve Overall Health*